HERBS FOR SINUS RELIEF

Harnessing Nature's Healing Power, Unlocking The Secrets Of Breathing Easy With Medicinal Solutions

DR. JEREMY ALLEY

Disclaimer:

The information provided in this book, is intended for general informational purposes only and should not be considered as professional advice.

The author has made every effort to ensure the accuracy of the information presented. However, readers are advised to consult with a qualified healthcare professional before attempting any herbal remedies or making significant changes to their wellness routine. Individual health conditions vary, and what may be suitable for one person may not be appropriate for another.

It is important to note that the author is not in any endorsement deal, partnership, or affiliation with any organization, brand, or company mentioned in this book. Any references to specific products or services are based on the author's personal experience or general knowledge and do not imply an endorsement or promotion of those products or services.

Contents

Overview

A long-lasting, continuous sinus irritation is the result of chronic sinusitis, a disorder that can greatly reduce a person's quality of life. This article attempts to investigate herbal medicines as a different method of treating persistent sinusitis, including considerations for people looking for natural remedies as well as insights into their possible advantages.

About This Book

The hallmark of chronic sinusitis, sometimes called chronic rhinosinusitis, is sinus inflammation that lasts for at least 12 weeks. In contrast to acute sinusitis, which is typically brought on by a viral or bacterial infection, chronic sinusitis is characterized by persistent inflammation that could be caused by several different things. Comprehending the characteristics of persistent sinusitis is essential to investigate efficacious herbal remedies that tackle its fundamental reasons.

Meaning and Signs

Acute sinusitis is not the only condition that can be defined as chronic sinusitis. It causes enduring symptoms such as thick mucus flow, facial pain or pressure, and congestion in the nose. The symptoms can greatly affect a person's everyday activities and range in intensity. A thorough study of these symptoms and how they relate to the underlying inflammatory processes is necessary to investigate herbal therapies.

Reasons and Danger Elements

Investigating the underlying causes and risk factors of chronic sinusitis is crucial to using herbal treatments to treat it effectively. Chronic sinusitis can arise and persist due to various factors, including allergies, deviated septum, nasal polyps, and respiratory infections. Herbal remedies can be customized to offer focused relief and support long-term sinus health by recognizing and treating these underlying causes.

Traditional Interventions and Restrictions

Conventional therapies for persistent sinusitis often entail the use of antibiotics, steroids, and decongestants; however, these may have drawbacks, including the possibility of repeated infections and adverse effects. Examining herbal medicines provides an alternate viewpoint by taking into account the possible advantages of organic substances with anti-inflammatory, antibacterial, and immune-modulating capabilities. Recognizing the shortcomings of traditional therapies paves the way for accepting herbal remedies as an adjunctive or substitute method of treating persistent sinusitis.

CHAPTER ONE

HERBAL MEDICATION FOR SINUOUS HEALTH

It can be difficult to treat chronic sinusitis, a condition marked by sinus inflammation that lasts longer than 12 weeks. While decongestants, steroids, and antibiotics are frequently used in traditional treatment, more people are turning to herbal therapies to relieve the symptoms and improve overall sinus health.

Herbal Remedies' Benefits

Herbal treatments for persistent sinusitis provide several advantages over prescription drugs. Their inherent therapeutic qualities, which come from plant-based substances utilized for ages in traditional medicine, are one obvious benefit. Herbal medicines usually have fewer negative effects than some pharmaceutical options, which makes them a desirable option for people looking for healing without unintended consequences. Herbal remedies also target the underlying causes of sinus problems in addition to their symptoms, which is in line with the holistic approach to well-being.

Organic Healing Capabilities

Reputable for their inherent medicinal qualities, herbs are essential for treating chronic sinusitis. For example, eucalyptus is well-known for its decongestant and anti-inflammatory properties. Clearing nasal passages and reducing sinus pressure can be achieved by inhaling steam infused with eucalyptus oil.

Another herb that is often used to treat infections linked to chronic sinusitis is goldenseal, which also has immune-stimulating and antibacterial qualities. Butterbur herb has also demonstrated potential in relieving symptoms such as headaches and congestion in the nose.

Very Few Side Effects

The low incidence of adverse effects is one of the main benefits of using herbal treatments to treat chronic sinusitis. Numerous prescription drugs used to treat sinusitis might have side effects like nausea, sleepiness, or other unpleasant side effects. Herbal treatments, on the other hand, frequently have fewer adverse effects, encouraging a kinder and more bearable approach to sinus health. Individual sensitivities can vary, so it's important to speak with a healthcare provider before introducing herbal therapies into a regimen.

A Comprehensive Approach To Wellbeing

Herbal medicines' holistic approach to well-being is consistent with the expanding notion that health is a complex system with many interconnected parts. Herbal remedies for chronic sinusitis take the patient's general health into account rather than just treating the symptoms. This method includes herbal remedies in addition to food recommendations, stress reduction techniques, and lifestyle factors. Herbal treatments add to a more thorough and long-lasting approach to treating chronic sinusitis by addressing the underlying causes and bolstering the body's natural healing processes.

Finally, for those with persistent sinusitis, the herbal approach to sinus health presents a strong alternative.

Herbal medicines are an appealing option because of their natural therapeutic qualities, low side effects, and holistic approach to wellness. To make sure that herbal remedies are appropriate for a person's needs and situations, it is crucial to speak with a healthcare provider before making any decisions about their health.

CHAPTER TWO

COMMON HERBS FOR THE RELIEF OF SINUS

A persistent and uncomfortable illness, chronic sinusitis frequently necessitates thorough and long-term remedies. Many people look into using herbal remedies in addition to or instead of traditional medical treatments. This section explores the characteristics and applications of common herbs that are well-known for their ability to effectively relieve chronic sinusitis.

Eucalyptus

Among the potent herbs, eucalyptus is particularly noteworthy for its benefits to sinus health. Some of its main ingredients, such as eucalyptol, have decongestant and anti-inflammatory properties. There are several ways to include eucalyptus in your sinus care regimen, and one of them is to make your own DIY eucalyptus steam inhalation.

This method is steam inhalation after a few drops of eucalyptus oil are added to boiling water. Inhaling steam soaked with eucalyptus oil can help relieve sinus pressure, lessen inflammation, and open up nasal passages.

Mint Pepper

Another plant with cooling and decongestant properties is peppermint, which makes it a useful ally when trying to relieve nasal congestion.

The menthol in peppermint helps relieve congestion by helping to widen the nasal passageways.

Including peppermint in your routine can be as easy as drinking peppermint tea, which has the added benefit of relieving sinus congestion and making for a calming and cozy brew. Over time, regular use of peppermint tea may help manage the symptoms of chronic sinusitis.

Ginger

Turmeric, well known for its strong anti-inflammatory qualities, has become an important component of herbal treatments for persistent sinusitis.

Curcumin, the main ingredient in turmeric, has been researched for its potential to lessen sinus-related discomfort and inflammation. Making a turmeric golden milk dish is one well-liked method to add turmeric to your diet.

Turmeric is combined with milk and honey to create a warm, soothing beverage that is both delicious and healthy, making it a great choice for anyone looking for all-natural remedies for chronic sinusitis.

By investigating these popular herbs for sinus relief, people can manage the symptoms of chronic sinusitis holistically.

Including these herbs in one's everyday routine—through inhaling steam, making herbal teas, or preparing dishes—can support a more all-encompassing and organic strategy for maintaining sinus health.

Before beginning any new herbal regimen, it is imperative to speak with a healthcare provider, particularly if you are taking medication or have pre-existing health conditions.

CHAPTER THREE

HERBAL TEAS FOR SUPPORTING SINUS

Herbal teas have long been valued for their medicinal qualities, providing a safe and natural remedy for a range of illnesses, including sinusitis. Of all the teas, chamomile and ginger tea are particularly notable for their potential to reduce inflammation and offer relief.

Tea with Chamomile

The Matricaria chamomilla plant yields chamomile, which is well known for its sedative and anti-inflammatory qualities. These characteristics make chamomile tea a possible ally for people who suffer from persistent sinusitis. Chamomile tea may help with less congestion and better breathing by reducing inflammation in the sinus passages. A program that includes regular chamomile tea consumption might be a gentle yet effective way to manage sinusitis.

Reducing Inflammation

It is believed that substances like bisabolol and chamazulene are responsible for chamomile's anti-inflammatory qualities. Together, these elements lessen inflammation and encourage a calming impact on inflamed nasal tissues. People may have less sinus pressure and congestion when the inflammation goes down, which will improve comfort.

The Right Brewing Methods

Caution when boiling chamomile tea is essential to maximizing its health benefits. Infuse one or two tablespoons of dried chamomile flowers in boiling water for five to ten minutes. This permits the release of active ingredients and essential oils. Several times a day, especially during flare-ups, brewing this tea could help manage chronic sinusitis more comprehensively.

Tea with Ginger

With a long history of use in traditional medicine, ginger is a multipurpose herb with strong anti-inflammatory and antioxidant qualities. Because of these benefits, ginger tea is a very attractive option for people looking for natural treatments for persistent sinusitis.

Properties Of Antioxidants

The efficacy of ginger's antioxidants, especially gingerol, to reduce inflammation and oxidative stress has been researched. Ginger tea may help to lessen the persistent inflammation that is frequently associated with chronic sinusitis. Ginger tea has the potential to reduce sinus problems by reducing inflammation and counteracting free radicals.

Infusion with Ginger and Lemon

Lemon enhances the health benefits of ginger tea by adding a pleasant touch and supplying extra vitamin C, which boosts the immune system. This injection offers a comprehensive approach to sinus health in addition to satisfying palates. Ginger and lemon together may aid in the breakdown of mucus, relieving congestion and encouraging sinus outflow.

Finally, for those suffering from chronic sinusitis, herbal medicines like chamomile and ginger tea present intriguing options. Incorporating these natural remedies into a thorough sinus care regimen may alleviate symptoms and improve general health. Before making any big changes to your health regimen, as with any other, it's best to speak with a healthcare provider, especially if you have any underlying medical concerns or are on prescription drugs.

CHAPTER FOUR

ESSENTIAL OILS FOR REMEDY OF SINUX

People who have chronic sinusitis, which is defined by ongoing inflammation of the sinus passages, frequently look for treatment for their condition through alternative therapies. The potential therapeutic effects of essential oils in reducing sinus congestion and discomfort have led to a rise in their popularity. Tea Tree Oil is a very strong option among these oils.

Tea Tree Liquid

Due to its well-known antifungal and antibacterial qualities, tea tree oil is a useful tool in the fight against sinus infections. Because of its inherent antibacterial properties, it can help get rid of fungi and bacteria that could be causing your sinusitis symptoms. DIY inhalation is one of the common ways that Tea Tree Oil is incorporated into sinus relief regimens.

Advantages Of Antifungal And Antibacterial

For those looking for natural treatments for chronic sinusitis, tea tree oil is an attractive option due to its antifungal and antibacterial properties.

Because of the oil's capacity to identify and eradicate dangerous microorganisms, sinus inflammation may be lessened and general sinus health may be enhanced. This makes it a flexible choice for people wishing to use herbal remedies in addition to conventional ones.

DIY Inhalation of Tea Tree Oil

DIY inhalation methods are one common way that people use tea tree oil to relieve sinus congestion. One way to feel better is to add a few drops of Tea Tree Oil to a bowl of hot water and inhale the steam, which helps clear sinus congestion. By using this method, the fragrant qualities of the oil can enter the respiratory system and relieve sore sinuses.

Oil of Lavender

Lavender oil is another essential oil that shows potential in treating chronic sinusitis. Lavender oil is known for its relaxing and aromatic qualities, but it can also help soothe sinus inflammation and support respiratory health in general.

Relieving Sinus Pain

The soothing effects of lavender oil also relieve sinus irritation, which helps people who are in pain from persistent sinusitis.

Breathing in the calming aroma of lavender oil can help promote relaxation and ease the stress and pain that come with ongoing sinus problems.

Techniques For Diffusion Of Lavender Oil

The benefits of lavender oil for sinus relief can be continuously and conveniently experienced by incorporating it into daily activities through diffusion techniques. Popular techniques include using essential oil diffusers or adding a few drops to a bowl of hot water for steam inhalation. Diffusing lavender oil throughout the house can help to produce a sinus-comforting environment, which is why it's a popular herbal cure for people with persistent sinusitis.

Before adding essential oils to a treatment plan, like with any herbal cure, it is imperative to speak with a healthcare provider, particularly for people with pre-existing medical issues or those on prescribed medication. An all-encompassing strategy for treating chronic sinusitis can include an awareness of the possible advantages and disadvantages of using herbal medicines.

CHAPTER FIVE

HERBAL TINCTURES AND SUPPLEMENTS

When treating chronic sinusitis, which is characterized by persistent sinus inflammation, a holistic approach is frequently necessary to minimize symptoms. The promise of herbal remedies and tinctures to relieve chronic sinusitis has led to their increasing popularity. The primary goals of these natural treatments are to treat the underlying issues and enhance general sinus health.

Extract From Butterbur

A well-known herbal treatment for persistent sinusitis is extract from butterbur. The scientific name for butterbur is Petasites hybridus, and it has been used traditionally for a variety of medical uses. Its root extract is a promising treatment option for sinus-related conditions since it contains active ingredients with anti-inflammatory qualities.

Including Butterbur extract in your regimen for treating sinusitis may help to lower inflammation and ease symptoms.

Handling Headaches

One typical and bothersome sign of chronic sinusitis is sinus headaches. An all-natural method of treating these headaches is provided by herbal treatments. Many herbs have been used for their analgesic and anti-inflammatory qualities, including willow bark and feverfew. Making herbal teas or using these plants in your regular regimen could help ease sinus headaches and improve general health.

Suggested Dosage

It is important to use herbal supplements such as butterbur extract according to approved dosages. Speaking with a healthcare provider or herbalist can help you receive individualized advice depending on your needs and state of health. A correct dosage guarantees that you won't experience any negative reactions or side effects while still benefiting from the herbal remedy's therapeutic properties.

Echinacea

Another herbal medicine that may help maintain sinus health is echinacea. Echinacea, which is well-known for boosting immunity, can aid the body in warding off infections that could lead to chronic sinusitis. Including echinacea in your diet, through supplements or herbal teas, can strengthen your body's defenses against illness.

Increasing Immune Function

Boosting the immune system is essential for treating chronic sinusitis. Astragalus and goldenseal are two well-known herbal supplements that are known to strengthen the immune system. By adding these herbs to your daily routine, you can strengthen your immune system continuously and lower your risk of sinus infections again.

Including Echinacea in Everyday Activities

It is necessary to regularly include echinacea in your daily routine to reap the full benefits of this plant.

There are several ways to accomplish this, including using tinctures, herbal teas, or supplements containing echinacea.

Frequent consumption guarantees a steady supply of immune-boosting substances, assisting your body in keeping its resistance against sinus-related problems.

Herbal treatments provide a safe, all-natural method of treating persistent sinusitis. These herbs, which vary from Echinacea to butterbur extract, have several advantages, such as analgesic, immune-stimulating, and anti-inflammatory qualities.

It is important to speak with medical professionals when thinking about using herbal supplements to figure out the right dosage for your unique requirements. By including these herbal therapies in your daily routine, you may be able to promote overall sinus health and achieve long-term relief from the symptoms of chronic sinusitis.

CHAPTER SIX

SUGGESTIONS FOR DIET IN SINUS HEALTH

Keeping up a balanced diet is crucial to treating persistent sinusitis. The foods we eat have a big impact on whether sinus problems get better or worse. In particular, an anti-inflammatory diet can play a significant role in lowering inflammation and improving sinus health in general.

a diet low in inflammation

Foods To Add

Adding items that reduce inflammation to one's diet is essential for those who have chronic sinusitis. These meals can reduce inflammation and regulate the immune system. Fish high in omega-3 fatty acids, such as mackerel and salmon, can be helpful. Furthermore, berries, cherries, and leafy greens are examples of fruits and vegetables strong in antioxidants that can help reduce inflammation.

Items To Steer Clear Of

Some foods have the potential to exacerbate sinus symptoms by causing inflammation. For example, dairy products may cause an increase in mucus production, which exacerbates congestion. Foods that have been processed and are heavy in preservatives and additives can also cause inflammatory reactions. People who suffer from persistent sinusitis ought to think about consuming fewer of these possibly irritating foods.

Hydration and Support for the Sinuses

The Value Of Adequate Hydration

Maintaining proper hydration is essential for good health in general and becomes more crucial when treating chronic sinusitis. Maintaining the thin consistency of nasal mucus with proper hydration helps avoid congestion and makes breathing easier. Additionally, it helps the body's natural detoxification processes by removing germs and allergens.

Herbal Drinks To Stay Hydrated

Herbal infusions can provide focused assistance for sinus health in addition to plain water. Some herbs can reduce inflammation and encourage nasal discharge.

For instance, peppermint tea is well-known for its decongestant qualities, which help to relieve nasal congestion.

In a similar vein, the anti-inflammatory properties of chamomile tea can help reduce sinus inflammation. Adding these herbal infusions to regular hydration regimens can support conventional treatments for persistent sinusitis.

Managing chronic sinusitis requires a comprehensive approach to dietary choices, emphasizing anti-inflammatory foods and making sure you are properly hydrated with herbal infusions. These lifestyle changes can help promote better sinus health and general well-being, especially when paired with further medical interventions as needed.

CHAPTER SEVEN

LIFESTYLE MODIFICATIONS TO PREVENT SINUSITIS

The cornerstone of treating chronic sinusitis is implementing a healthy lifestyle. This section looks at a variety of routines and practices that can help avoid sinus problems. Beyond using herbal medicines, readers will learn about holistic techniques that take into account environmental elements and dietary issues.

Nasal Irrigation: Advantages And Methods

Nasal irrigation is one of the main natural treatments for persistent sinusitis. The advantages of this practice are covered in this subsection, with special attention to how well it clears the nasal passages of allergens, irritants, and excess mucus. Readers can choose the best method for adding nasal irrigation to their daily practice by investigating various approaches.

Make Your Own Saline Solutions

Homemade saline solutions are an affordable, natural alternative in the field of nasal irrigation. This section of the book explains how people can make their saline solutions at home, giving them complete control over the components and the ability to customize the solution to meet their own needs. By being aware of the ingredients and methods for making DIY saline solutions, readers may take control of their sinus health.

Stress Reduction

Stress has a significant effect on sinus health as well as general health. This section delves into the complex relationship between chronic sinusitis and stress, highlighting the critical impact that stress management can have in reducing symptoms.

There is a discussion of herbal remedies for stress alleviation, giving readers comprehensive methods to improve their general health and lessen the negative effects of stress on sinus health.

Techniques For Relaxation

Using relaxation techniques is crucial while trying to treat chronic sinusitis. This part explores a variety of herbal and non-herbal relaxation techniques that can help induce calmness and lower stress levels. Readers will learn about many methods to improve their sinus health and promote relaxation, ranging from mindfulness exercises to herbal teas.

CHAPTER EIGHT

THE ESSENTIAL MEDICINE'S POWER

Herbal medicine recognizes that plants can treat a wide range of illnesses and uses these qualities to its advantage. Herbs such as echinacea, butterbur, and goldenseal are popular choices for treating chronic sinusitis because of their immune-stimulating and anti-inflammatory properties. These herbs might help lessen nasal inflammation and stop infections from happening again.

Safety Factors

Safety considerations must be taken into account before adding herbal therapies to a sinusitis treatment strategy. Not every person can use herbs, and it's important to consider any conflicts with drugs or underlying medical issues.

It is best to speak with a healthcare provider or herbalist to make sure that the herbs selected fit the health profile of the client.

Selecting The Correct Herbs For Clear Sinuses

A key component of using herbs as a remedy for chronic sinusitis is choosing the right herbs. Congestion may be reduced by using saline solutions infused with herbs, such as peppermint oil or eucalyptus, via nasal irrigation.

Herbal teas that contain substances like licorice root, ginger, and chamomile may also have calming effects on sinus symptoms.

CHAPTER NINE

CASE RESEARCH

Real-world case studies are among the most enlightening ways to comprehend the efficacy of herbal therapies for persistent sinusitis. These testimonies offer insight into the lives of those who have included herbal remedies in their regimen. By looking at these examples, we can find trends, obstacles, and solutions for managing chronic sinusitis with herbs.

Achievement Stories

Success stories are a source of encouragement for anyone struggling with the intricacies of persistent sinusitis. This section features people who have used herbal medicines consistently and not only had symptom relief but also a notable increase in their general well-being. These success stories are meant to encourage and direct others toward improved health.

Every person has a different path to wellness, and personal experiences can offer important insights into the difficulties and victories encountered when trying to find treatment for persistent sinusitis. Through the sharing of these personal accounts, this section hopes to establish a stronger emotional connection with readers by providing relatable stories and useful advice that can support them on their path to better sinus health.

We will explore the several plants, herbs, and natural methods that have demonstrated potential in treating the symptoms of chronic sinusitis as we delve into the rich field of herbal medicines.

This investigation attempts to provide you with the information and understanding necessary to make wise decisions regarding the health of your sinuses, regardless of whether you are looking for complementary or alternative therapies.

VERDICT

While reviewing herbal remedies for chronic sinusitis, keep in mind that each person's reaction may be different. Herbal therapies may provide symptom alleviation for some people, but other people may not benefit in the same way. Patience and consistency in use are essential because herbal remedies sometimes take some time to show results.

Promotion Of A Holistic Way Of Living

Adopting a holistic lifestyle is just as crucial for managing chronic sinusitis as herbal medicines. This includes eating a balanced diet, drinking plenty of water, cleaning your nose properly, and controlling your stress.

Holistic methods take into account a person's whole well-being, which makes them more all-encompassing and long-lasting when it comes to sinus health.

Herbal treatments might be a useful complement to conventional sinusitis treatment. But it's important to approach these treatments mindfully and cautiously, taking into account each patient's unique medical situation. Herbal treatments combined with a holistic lifestyle could provide a more comprehensive approach for people looking for natural ways to relieve long-term sinusitis problems.